Acne Diet Plan

A Beginner's Step-by-Step Guide to Managing Acne Through Nutrition With Curated Recipes and a Sample Meal Plan

mf

copyright © 2024 Brandon Gilta

All rights reserved No part of this book may be reproduced, or stored in a retrieval system, or transmitted in any form or by any means, electronic, mechanical, photocopying, recording, or otherwise, without express written permission of the publisher.

Disclaimer

By reading this disclaimer, you are accepting the terms of the disclaimer in full. If you disagree with this disclaimer, please do not read the guide.

All of the content within this guide is provided for informational and educational purposes only, and should not be accepted as independent medical or other professional advice. The author is not a doctor, physician, nurse, mental health provider, or registered nutritionist/dietician. Therefore, using and reading this guide does not establish any form of a physician-patient relationship.

Always consult with a physician or another qualified health provider with any issues or questions you might have regarding any sort of medical condition. Do not ever disregard any qualified professional medical advice or delay seeking that advice because of anything you have read in this guide. The information in this guide is not intended to be any sort of medical advice and should not be used in lieu of any medical advice by a licensed and qualified medical professional.

The information in this guide has been compiled from a variety of known sources. However, the author cannot attest to or guarantee the accuracy of each source and thus should not be held liable for any errors or omissions.

You acknowledge that the publisher of this guide will not be held liable for any loss or damage of any kind incurred as a result of this guide or the reliance on any information provided within this guide. You acknowledge and agree that you assume all risk and responsibility for any action you undertake in response to the information in this guide.

Using this guide does not guarantee any particular result (e.g., weight loss or a cure). By reading this guide, you acknowledge that there are no guarantees to any specific outcome or results you can expect.

All product names, diet plans, or names used in this guide are for identification purposes only and are the property of their respective owners. The use of these names does not imply endorsement. All other trademarks cited herein are the property of their respective owners.

Where applicable, this guide is not intended to be a substitute for the original work of this diet plan and is, at most, a supplement to the original work for this diet plan and never a direct substitute. This guide is a personal expression of the facts of that diet plan.

Where applicable, persons shown in the cover images are stock photography models and the publisher has obtained the rights to use the images through license agreements with third-party stock image companies.

Table of Contents

Introduction — 8
Understanding Acne — 11
   It's All Acne, Actually — 11
   Causes of Acne — 13
   Symptoms of Acne — 14
   Treatment for Acne — 15
   Types of Acne Treatment — 16
   Friends of Your Face — 19
   Oral medications — 20
   Lifestyle Changes to Manage Acne — 20

What Is Acne Diet? — 23
   Principles of Acne Diet — 23
   Benefits of Acne Diet — 25
   Disadvantages of Acne Diet — 26

A 5-Step Guide to Getting Started with the Acne Diet — 28
   Step 1: Understand the Connection Between Diet and Acne — 28
   Step 2: Identify Acne-Triggering Foods — 29
   Step 3: Plan Your Acne Diet — 31
   Step 4: Implement the Acne Diet — 32
   Step 5: Monitor Your Progress — 34
   Foods to Eat — 35

Sample Meal Plan — 38
   Day 1 — 38
   Day 2 — 38
   Day 3 — 39
   Day 4 — 40
   Day 5 — 40
   Day 6 — 41
   Day 7 — 41

Sample Recipes — 43
- Baked Mackerel with Sweet Potato and Kale Salad — 44
- Salmon Steak and Cauliflower Mash — 46
- Avocado, Cucumber, and Tomato Salad — 48
- Honey Chicken and Avocado Salad — 50
- Veggie Omelet — 52
- Baked Almond Chicken with Cherry and Balsamic — 54
- Blueberry Flax Smoothie — 56
- Grilled Chicken and Mushrooms — 57
- Energy Oats — 59
- Fresh Cucumber Salad — 61
- Baked Salmon with Garlic and Dijon Dressing — 62
- Mediterranean Breakfast — 63
- One-pot beans and Zucchini Penne — 65
- Baked Tuna and Asparagus — 67
- Avocado Spinach Smoothie — 69
- Quinoa Salad with Salmon and Veggies — 70
- Sweet Potato and Black Bean Tacos — 72
- Blueberry Almond Overnight Oats — 74
- Green Tea Matcha Smoothie — 75
- Turmeric and Ginger Stir-Fry — 76

Conclusion — 78
FAQ — 82
References and Helpful Links — 84

Introduction

Acne - a condition often tied to teenage years, skin concerns, and an ongoing search for effective remedies. This prevalent skin issue doesn't only affect teenagers, but individuals of various age groups worldwide. A potential solution to this enduring problem doesn't always have to involve high-end creams or harsh treatments. It could be as simple as adjusting your dietary habits. This introduces us to the concept of the Acne Diet Plan.

The link between diet and acne has been a subject of discussion for decades. However, recent scientific studies suggest that the food you consume can indeed influence your skin health. It's key to note that no single food directly causes or cures acne; nevertheless, certain dietary habits can either exacerbate or alleviate its severity. Here's where the Acne Diet Plan becomes relevant, offering a complete guide to how your nutrition can impact your skin's health.

Clear, radiant skin can contribute to self-confidence and overall well-being. The Acne Diet Plan presents an opportunity to work towards these benefits. This plan isn't a quick fix but a sustainable lifestyle change that could significantly improve your skin's health and appearance. Furthermore, this plan extends beyond just tackling acne; it also encourages overall wellness, potentially leading to enhanced energy levels, improved digestion, and a better mood.

In this guide, we will talk about the following;

- All about acne, its different types, and its possible causes
- Different modes of treatment, depending on the severity of the case, and the different ingredients or chemicals used for the treatment and prevention of acne
- Step-by-step guide to get started with acne diet
- The controversy between diet and acne, foods to avoid, and foods to embrace
- Sample acne-clearing recipes for you to try
- Sample meals for 7 days to kick start you into a healthier, clearer skin diet

If you're prepared to take control of your skin health and are open to making dietary changes that could contribute to clearer, healthier skin, then continue reading this guide. We will explore the specifics of the Acne Diet Plan, providing a detailed understanding of the foods to limit and those to include, and how these dietary adjustments can aid in managing your acne.

Armed with a week-long sample meal plan and tips on additional lifestyle changes that complement the diet, you'll be ready to start this journey towards clear skin. By sticking to the Acne Diet Plan, you're not just working towards healthier skin but also incorporating better eating habits that can enhance your overall well-being. It's time to move beyond acne and embrace a healthier, more confident version of yourself.

Keep reading as we deepen our understanding of the Acne Diet Plan—a comprehensive guide to managing acne from within. Your journey towards clearer skin starts here.

Understanding Acne

Acne, or *acne vulgaris*, is a skin disease caused by clogged hair follicles. Hair follicles can get clogged by oil naturally produced by the body, or by dead skin cells. Sometimes, it's caused by bacteria or fungi as well.

One of the common misconceptions is that acne only refers to the inflamed, pus-filled bumps on the face or back; it doesn't. Acne includes not only what you'd call pimples or zits, but also blackheads, whiteheads, and cysts.

Another common misconception is that acne only pops up on a person's face and back. Technically, any hair follicle along the skin can get clogged up and therefore cause acne, but it most often happens in areas where oil production is high. So, yes, it occurs mostly in the face and back, but it can also appear in the chest, neck, and even around the pelvis and buttocks.

It's All Acne, Actually

Yes, the small bumps dotting your face and the small black spots are also acne. They're known as whiteheads and blackheads, but the proper scientific term for both is comedones.

Comedones are clogged pores or hair follicles. Both "versions" of comedones are clogged up by oil, dead skin cells, or a combination of both. The difference between the two is that whiteheads are closed comedones while blackheads are open. Open comedones turn black because the gunk inside oxidizes once exposed to air.

Pimples or zits are also comedones like whiteheads and blackheads. When the clog gets infected by bacteria, the comedo (the singular form of comedones) gets inflamed and filled with pus. Inflamed, pus-filled comedones are called pustules.

In some cases, pustules form deeper into the skin's layer. This results in a painful lump colloquially called "cysts." They're not true cysts, however, and are technically nodules.

Most cases of acne are a combination of some or even all of these. Unfortunately, there are no globally accepted criteria for classifying mild, moderate, and severe acne, so it's usually up to the discretion of the dermatologist. It's widely accepted that mild acne refers to comedones, or whiteheads and blackheads, that appear occasionally only on the face. Moderate acne is when there's a noticeable number of pimples, or inflamed, pus-filled pustules. The pimples might also appear on the back and chest area. Lastly, severe acne is when there are nodules on the face and chest.

Aside from comedones, acne almost always presents in people with oily skin. There's also scarring and hyperpigmentation involved in almost all cases.

Causes of Acne

Acne, a common skin condition, can be caused by a variety of factors. Each cause contributes in its own way to the development of breakouts. Here are some key causes:

- **Hormonal Changes**: During certain stages of life like puberty or pregnancy, our bodies experience hormonal fluctuations. These changes can stimulate the sebaceous glands to produce more oil, leading to clogged pores and acne.
- **Poor Diet**: Consuming foods high in refined sugars or dairy products may trigger acne in some individuals. These foods can cause inflammation and spike blood sugar levels, contributing to breakouts.
- **Stress**: High stress levels can cause the body to produce hormones such as cortisol, which can stimulate oil production in the skin and lead to acne.
- **Certain Medications**: Some drugs, including certain types of steroids, lithium, or hormonal medications, can cause acne as a side effect. They can alter the body's hormone levels or cause changes in the skin.

- **Poor Hygiene**: Not cleaning the skin properly or regularly can lead to the buildup of oils and dead skin cells. This can clog pores, providing a breeding ground for bacteria and leading to acne.
- **Genetics**: If your parents had acne, you're more likely to have it too. Genetic factors can make some people more prone to getting acne and having more severe breakouts.

Each of these causes plays a role in the onset of acne, and understanding them is the first step towards effective treatment and prevention."

Symptoms of Acne

Acne is not just about having pimples; it presents itself in a variety of symptoms, each with its unique characteristics. Here are some of the most common symptoms:

- **Whiteheads**: These are clogged pores that have closed up. They appear as small, white bumps on the skin's surface caused by the accumulation of oil and dead skin cells.
- **Blackheads**: These are clogged pores that remain open. The black color is not due to dirt but rather the oxidation of the trapped substances when exposed to air.

- **Papules**: These are small, red, and tender bumps on the skin. They occur when the walls surrounding your skin pores break down due to severe inflammation.
- **Pustules**: These are similar to papules but contain pus. They appear as red bumps with white or yellow tips and are a result of an infection in the hair follicle.
- **Nodules**: These are substantial, firm, and discomforting bumps that reside underneath the skin's surface. They occur due to the accumulation of secretions deep inside the hair follicles.
- **Cysts**: These are painful, pus-filled lumps beneath the skin's surface. They form when the infection leads to a rupture in the walls of the pore, causing severe inflammation.

Identifying these symptoms is crucial to determining the severity of acne and deciding the most effective treatment approach.

Treatment for Acne

So, now that we know what acne is and what causes it, how do you stop it?

Preventing and treating acne will rely on controlling the cause. For example, if your acne is caused by dead skin cells and sebum, your acne will get better if you use products that will speed up the sloughing of dead skin cells and products that control sebum. If your acne is caused by hormones, taking hormone therapy will help. If your acne is caused by bacteria, a round of antibiotics will treat it.

Types of Acne Treatment

The treatment of acne depends on the severity and cause. Mild to moderate cases can be treated by topical and over-the-counter medications, but the more severe forms can require prescription medicines and even surgery.

The three common kinds of treatment are the following:

- Topical treatments
- Oral medications
- Surgery

Let's take a brief look at each of them.

Topical treatments

Topical treatments are the most common of the three. They include creams, ointments, and other skincare items that target acne caused by clogging and, to an extent, bacteria.

It is interesting to note that Western skincare is somewhat different than Asian skincare, in that most Western skincare products are formulated to treat existing acne while Asian skincare is meant to prevent it. For example, most Western skincare products for acne have active ingredients that aim to treat existing acne, while Asian skincare aims to balance the skin, therefore preventing breakouts.

Most Western skincare products for acne tend to be astringent, harsher, and dry to the skin. This is because it's an immediate form of oil control. On the other hand, Asian skincare products are milder, to balance the skin by keeping it hydrated and moisturized.

This isn't to say that one is inherently better than the other. You might find that a mix of the two might be best for your skin.

Oral Medications

Oral medications are usually given to people suffering from acne caused by bacteria, or from acne caused by a hormone imbalance. Oral medications include antibiotics, anti-androgen medications, and even contraceptive pills.

Some of these medicines are over-the-counter, but it's best to consult a dermatologist before taking any medications.

Some oral medicines are stronger types of antibiotics that will require a doctor's prescription. These are usually reserved for the more severe cases of acne, however.

Surgery

People with severe and painful closed comedones might find it challenging to treat their acne with non-invasive methods alone. The term "surgery" can sound daunting, but most surgical procedures for acne are straightforward and performed on an outpatient basis. Here are some of the most common surgical treatments for acne:

- Excision: This is a common procedure where the dermatologist makes a small incision to open the clogged comedones, allowing the trapped pus and debris to be drained. Local anesthesia is typically used to ensure comfort during the procedure.
- Extraction: This is a routine procedure that can even be performed outside a clinical setting, such as in beauty spas. Licensed aestheticians carefully squeeze the comedones to remove the blockage.
- Chemical Peels: Ideal for mild to moderate acne, this procedure involves applying a type of acid to the skin to exfoliate the outer layers, revealing the closed comedones underneath and preventing new ones from forming. While mild chemical peels can be bought in drugstores, stronger versions that penetrate deeper skin layers should be administered by a dermatologist.
- Laser Surgery: This method can address acne caused by bacterial infections, as well as scarring and hyperpigmentation resulting from acne. Laser treatments usually require multiple sessions and can be costly.
- Intralesional Injections: These are shots of cortisone injected directly into the comedo. They're typically used for inflamed and painful pimples, which will flatten out a few hours after the injection. While

effective, this treatment serves as a temporary solution, and addressing the root cause of the acne is still necessary.

Remember, it's essential to consult with a healthcare provider or a dermatologist for professional advice before deciding on any treatment.

Friends of Your Face

Let's look at some ingredients or chemicals used to treat acne.

Topical treatments

One common ingredient is benzoyl peroxide. It's a chemical used for non-severe forms of acne. It has an antibacterial effect that also makes it effective against acne caused by bacteria. Many benzoyl peroxide preparations are mixed with another chemical or antibiotic, like clindamycin or salicylic acid.

Salicylic acid is another acne treatment. It might sound dangerous, but it's a mild acid that penetrates deeper into the pores or hair follicles and melts the gunk inside. It also helps in exfoliating the skin. This makes it effective in treating blackheads. Salicylic acid is used in varying strengths for chemical peels.

Another ingredient is AHA or alpha hydroxy acid. It's another gentle type of acid that works best at exfoliating the outer layers of the skin, making it a great treatment or preventive measure against whiteheads.

Severe nodular acne requires a more targeted type of treatment. The medicines used for it require a prescription in most countries. The most common treatment for it is tretinoin, a retinoid with strong astringent properties. It promotes rapid skill cell turnover and sebum control. However, too strong a dose can cause severe burns and photosensitivity.

Tretinoin and other derivatives of retinoids can also be found in topical creams and gels.

Oral medications

Hormonal acne responds best to hormonal therapy. The most common of these are anti-androgen medicines (for men) or oral contraceptives (for women). Because hormones and experienced side effects vary from person to person, you might need to cycle through several pills before you find the formulation that works best with you.

A type of tretinoin, isotretinoin, is an oral medication used to treat severe acne.

Lifestyle Changes to Manage Acne

Managing acne often involves making certain lifestyle changes that can help reduce breakouts and improve overall skin health. Some of these changes include:

- **Maintaining a Balanced Diet**: A diet rich in fruits, vegetables, lean proteins, and whole grains promotes overall health and can potentially help manage acne. While the link between diet and acne isn't definitive, some research suggests that food with a high glycemic index could trigger breakouts. Therefore, limiting processed foods and sugary drinks may benefit those with acne-prone skin.
- **Regular Exercise**: Regular physical activity helps increase blood circulation, reducing stress and promoting healthy skin. However, it's crucial to shower after exercising, as sweat can clog pores and exacerbate acne.
- **Proper Hydration**: Drinking plenty of water helps maintain the skin's elasticity and can aid in detoxification, potentially reducing the occurrence of acne.
- **Adequate Sleep**: Quality sleep is vital for skin health. During sleep, the body repairs and regenerates skin cells, which can help manage acne.
- **Stress Management**: Chronic stress can worsen acne by triggering hormonal changes. Techniques such as yoga, meditation, and deep breathing can help manage stress levels and potentially reduce breakouts.
- **Good Skincare Routine**: Regularly washing the face, especially after sweating, using non-comedogenic products, and avoiding harsh scrubs can help manage

acne. It's also important not to pick or squeeze pimples, as this can lead to scarring and infection.

- **Limiting Sun Exposure**: While moderate sun exposure can benefit overall health, excessive exposure can irritate the skin and exacerbate acne. Using a non-comedogenic sunscreen and wearing protective clothing can help protect the skin.

Remember, everyone's skin reacts differently, and what works for one person might not work for another. It's always best to consult a dermatologist or healthcare provider before starting any new regimen to manage acne.

What Is Acne Diet?

Acne diet refers to a specific way of eating that is believed to help prevent or manage acne. It involves avoiding certain foods that may trigger acne breakouts and including others that are thought to have beneficial effects on the skin.

Before we dive into the details of an acne diet, it's important to note that there is no one-size-fits-all approach. Everyone's body is different and may react differently to certain foods. It's always best to consult with a healthcare professional before making significant changes to your diet. In the next section, we will discuss some principles, the benefits of an acne diet, and potential food triggers to avoid.

Principles of Acne Diet

The principles of an acne diet generally focus on consuming foods that promote skin health and avoiding those that may trigger or exacerbate acne. Here are some key principles:

- **Avoid High Glycemic Foods**: Foods with a high glycemic index can raise your blood sugar rapidly, leading to an insulin spike. This can result in inflammation and excess oil production, both of which can contribute to acne. High glycemic foods include processed snacks, sugary drinks, and white bread.

- **Consume Low-Glycemic Foods**: These are foods that don't cause a rapid rise in blood sugar levels. They include whole grains, legumes, fruits, and vegetables.
- **Limit Dairy Intake**: Some studies suggest a connection between dairy consumption and acne, possibly due to the hormones present in milk. While not everyone with acne needs to avoid dairy, those who notice a link between dairy consumption and their acne may benefit from limiting their intake.
- **Eat More Omega-3 Fatty Acids**: Foods rich in omega-3 fatty acids, like fish and flaxseeds, can help manage inflammation in the body, potentially reducing the severity of acne.
- **Stay Hydrated**: Drinking enough water can help keep your skin hydrated and may aid in the prevention of acne.
- **Consume Antioxidant-Rich Foods**: Antioxidants can help protect your skin from damage. Foods rich in antioxidants include berries, dark chocolate, and nuts.
- **Limit Processed Foods**: Processed foods often contain additives and preservatives that could aggravate acne.

Remember, everyone's skin is different, and what works for one person may not work for another. It's always a good idea to consult with a healthcare provider or a nutritionist before making major changes to your diet.

Benefits of Acne Diet

Adopting an acne diet can bring about numerous benefits, not just for your skin, but for your overall health as well. Here are some of the key benefits:

- **Reduced Inflammation**: A diet rich in anti-inflammatory foods like fruits, vegetables, and fatty fish can help reduce inflammation in the body, which in turn may decrease the severity of acne breakouts.
- **Balanced Blood Sugar Levels**: By limiting the intake of refined sugars and carbs, an acne diet helps maintain stable blood sugar levels. This can prevent insulin spikes that are linked to increased sebum production and acne.
- **Improved Gut Health**: Consuming probiotics and fiber-rich foods supports a healthy gut microbiome. A balanced gut can positively impact skin health and potentially help in managing acne.
- **Enhanced Skin Health**: Foods rich in vitamins A, E, and zinc contribute to skin health, aiding in cell turnover and reducing the likelihood of pores becoming clogged.

- **Healthy Weight Maintenance**: An acne diet typically emphasizes whole, nutrient-dense foods and limits processed items, which can also aid in maintaining a healthy weight.
- **Stress Management**: Certain foods, like those rich in antioxidants and omega-3 fatty acids, have been shown to help reduce stress levels. Since stress can trigger acne, a balanced diet can indirectly help manage breakouts.

Remember, while an acne diet can assist in managing symptoms, it should be combined with a proper skincare regimen for optimal results.

Disadvantages of Acne Diet

While an acne diet can be beneficial, it's not without its potential downsides. However, many find that the benefits outweigh these disadvantages. Here are some key points to consider:

- **Limited Food Choices**: An acne diet often implies avoiding certain foods like dairy products or those with a high glycemic index. This can limit food options and make meal planning more challenging.
- **Potential Nutrient Deficiencies**: If not properly managed, strict dietary modifications could lead to deficiencies in essential nutrients. For example, cutting out dairy might result in inadequate calcium intake.

- **Inconclusive Evidence**: While some people report improvements in their skin condition following an acne diet, there's no universal agreement in the scientific community on this.
- **Social Implications**: Sticking to an acne diet can be socially tricky, especially when dining out or attending social events where high-glycemic or dairy-rich foods are served.
- **Misconceptions about 'Greasy Foods'**: There's minimal proof to suggest that consuming oily foods directly leads to acne. It's the overactive oil-producing glands in the skin, not the dietary intake of fats and oils, that result in oily skin.

Despite these drawbacks, the potential benefits of an acne diet should not be dismissed. These include reduced inflammation, balanced blood sugar levels, improved gut health, enhanced skin health, healthy weight maintenance, and better stress management. Ultimately, it's about finding what works best for your body. Always consult with a healthcare professional before making drastic dietary changes.

A 5-Step Guide to Getting Started with the Acne Diet

Acne can be a stubborn problem, but did you know your diet could be a key factor in managing it? Let's explore a simple 5-step guide to help you get started with the ACNE diet.

Step 1: Understand the Connection Between Diet and Acne

The initial step in managing your skin health is to comprehend the profound connection between your diet and acne. It's vital to grasp that what you're fueling your body with can significantly affect your skin's appearance.

Scientific research has indicated that certain foods may contribute to acne breakouts. Specifically, foods high in sugar and saturated fats have been linked to triggering inflammation and hormonal imbalances in your body. These internal disruptions can manifest externally as acne breakouts.

When you consume a diet high in sugar, your body experiences a spike in insulin levels. This surge can lead to an overproduction of skin oils and cause a rapid cell turnover, both of which create a perfect environment for acne-causing bacteria to thrive. Similarly, foods high in unhealthy fats can also increase inflammation in your body, leading to potential skin eruptions.

On the other hand, making healthier food choices can have the opposite effect. A balanced diet rich in whole foods, fruits, vegetables, lean proteins, and healthy fats can help reduce inflammation and balance your hormones. As these internal systems reach equilibrium, you may find that your skin responds positively, with fewer breakouts and improved overall complexion.

Understanding this link between diet and skin health is crucial in your journey to clearer, healthier skin. By being mindful of your dietary choices, you're not only nourishing your body but also potentially lessening the occurrence of acne breakouts.

Step 2: Identify Acne-Triggering Foods

The subsequent step in your journey to clearer skin involves pinpointing the specific foods that might be exacerbating your acne. Some foods are notorious for their potential to contribute to breakouts, and taking a closer look at your diet can help in singling them out.

Dairy products, such as milk, cheese, and yogurt, are often linked to acne. While they can be a part of a healthy diet, these foods contain certain hormones that might lead to an imbalance in your own hormone levels, thereby triggering acne.

Processed foods, including fast food and packaged snacks, are also common culprits. They are often high in unhealthy fats and sugars, which can cause inflammation and lead to breakouts. Moreover, these foods lack the essential nutrients your skin needs to stay healthy, further contributing to skin issues.

Refined carbohydrates like white bread, pasta, and pastries can have a similar effect. These foods are quickly broken down into sugar in your body, leading to a surge in insulin levels. This spike can stimulate your skin to produce more oil, known as sebum, which can clog your pores and create an environment where acne-causing bacteria thrive.

Sugary drinks, such as sodas and certain fruit juices, are another category to watch out for. They can cause rapid spikes in your blood sugar levels, leading to increased sebum production and potentially resulting in clogged pores and breakouts.

Identifying these acne-triggering foods is not about completely eliminating them from your diet, but rather about understanding their effects on your skin and making more informed dietary choices. By being mindful of your intake of these foods and balancing them with healthier options, you can take a significant stride toward managing your acne.

Step 3: Plan Your Acne Diet

Armed with the knowledge of which foods could potentially trigger your acne, it's time to shift focus toward planning a skin-friendly diet. The goal here is not just about avoidance but about proactively including foods that can aid in reducing acne and promoting healthier skin.

Whole foods should be the cornerstone of your acne diet. These are foods that are unprocessed and unrefined, processed and refined as little as possible and are free from additives or other artificial substances. They are packed with essential nutrients that your body and skin need to function optimally.

Prioritize foods that are rich in antioxidants. Antioxidants help protect your skin from damage by neutralizing harmful free radicals in your body. Fruits like berries (strawberries, blueberries, raspberries) are excellent sources of antioxidants.

Incorporate vegetables, especially leafy greens like spinach and kale, into your diet. They are high in vitamins and minerals that can help reduce inflammation and keep your skin healthy.

Lean proteins, such as salmon and chicken, provide essential amino acids that your body needs to repair skin tissues.

Particularly, salmon is an excellent source of omega-3 fatty acids, known for their anti-inflammatory properties.

Whole grains like quinoa and brown rice are a better alternative to refined carbohydrates. They have a lower glycemic index, meaning they won't cause a sudden spike in your blood sugar levels, thus helping to regulate sebum production.

Lastly, don't forget about healthy fats. Foods like avocados and nuts contain monounsaturated and polyunsaturated fats that can keep your skin moisturized and supple, and help absorb vitamins that your skin needs.

Planning your acne diet is about creating a balanced and varied meal plan that supports your skin health. By making these nutritious foods a regular part of your diet, you're equipping your body with the tools it needs to fight off acne and promote healthier skin.

Step 4: Implement the Acne Diet

Now that you've planned your acne diet, the next step is to start incorporating it into your daily routine. This process isn't about abrupt changes or total deprivation, but rather about gradually introducing healthier alternatives into your meals.

Begin by identifying the acne-triggering foods in your current meal plan. Once you've pinpointed these, start replacing them with the skin-friendly options you've outlined in your acne diet. For instance, if you often have white bread for breakfast, consider switching to whole-grain bread. If you frequently indulge in sugary drinks, try substituting them with water or herbal tea.

Remember, this is not about completely eliminating the foods you love. It's perfectly fine to treat yourself occasionally. The goal is to make smarter choices most of the time. You can still enjoy your favorite foods but aim to balance them with nutritious options that benefit your skin.

Consistency plays a crucial role in this process. Implementing the acne diet is not a one-time event but a long-term commitment. It might take some time before you see significant changes in your skin's health. Don't be disheartened if you don't see immediate results. Skin regeneration takes time, and the positive effects of dietary changes tend to appear gradually.

Over time, these small dietary adjustments can accumulate substantial benefits for your skin health. Each healthy meal brings you one step closer to clearer, healthier skin. Remember, your food choices are powerful tools in managing acne, and with consistency and patience, you're likely to see progress.

Step 5: Monitor Your Progress

The final step in implementing your acne diet is to diligently monitor the changes in your skin. This involves observing and documenting how your skin responds to the dietary shifts you're making.

Start by taking note of your skin's condition before you begin the acne diet. You could even take a photograph for a visual record. This will provide a baseline against which you can compare future changes. As you progress with your diet, continue to document any noticeable changes in your skin's health. This could be a decrease in the number of breakouts, less redness, or an improvement in your skin's overall texture and tone.

Remember that improvements might not be immediate. It may take several weeks or even a few months to see significant changes. This is because your skin cells renew themselves approximately every 30 days, and it takes time for the benefits of your new diet to manifest in your skin's appearance. Therefore, patience and persistence are crucial during this period.

If, after several months, you don't see any improvements, or if your acne worsens, it might be time to seek professional help. A consultation with a dermatologist or a dietitian could provide you with personalized advice tailored to your specific needs and conditions. They can help identify any other potential triggers or underlying issues that may be contributing to your acne and guide you on the best course of action moving forward.

Monitoring your progress is not just about tracking improvements; it's also about learning how your body responds to different foods. This knowledge can empower you to make informed decisions about your diet and lifestyle, ultimately leading to healthier skin.

Foods to Eat

Maintaining clear, acne-free skin may be supported by a diet rich in omega-3 fatty acids, dietary fiber, and antioxidants. These nutrients can be found in a variety of foods and can provide numerous benefits for your skin health:

Omega-3 Fatty Acids

Omega-3s are known for their anti-inflammatory properties and may help alleviate the inflammation associated with acne breakouts. Foods high in omega-3 include:

- Fatty fish (e.g., sardines, salmon, mackerel)
- Soy products (e.g., tofu, soybeans)
- Eggs
- Leafy greens (e.g., kale, spinach)
- Grass-fed beef
- Nuts and seeds (e.g., almonds, flaxseed, walnuts)
- Wild rice

Dietary Fiber

Although the relationship between dietary fiber and acne is not entirely understood, fiber is believed to assist in waste elimination from the body, potentially helping to keep skin clear by regulating blood sugar levels. Foods rich in dietary fiber include:

- Fruits (e.g., apples, berries)
- Vegetables (e.g., carrots)
- Oatmeal
- Beans
- Corn
- Wholegrain cereals, bread, and pasta

Antioxidants

Antioxidants can help combat free radicals that can cause skin inflammation, collagen breakdown, and dark spots – all factors that can contribute to acne. A diverse diet can ensure a good intake of antioxidants. Foods abundant in antioxidants include:

- Strong-smelling vegetables (e.g., garlic, leeks, onions)
- Dark-colored fruits and vegetables (e.g., blueberries, eggplants, grapes)
- Beverages such as red wine and tea
- Seafood
- Cruciferous vegetables (e.g., broccoli, cauliflower, cabbage)

- Plant proteins (e.g., soybeans, lentils, tofu, peas)
- Healthy fats from avocados, nuts, and seeds
- Organ meats, especially liver
- Egg yolks
- Vitamin C-rich fruits (e.g., oranges, strawberries, mangoes, blackcurrants)

In summary, incorporating these foods into your diet may help manage acne by providing the nutrients your skin needs to stay healthy and clear.

Sample Meal Plan

Day 1

Breakfast

- Avocado toast on whole-grain bread
- Blueberries

Lunch

- Salmon steak and cauliflower mash

Dinner

- Baked salmon with a side of steamed broccoli and wild rice

Snacks

- Almonds
- Apple

Day 2

Breakfast

- Oatmeal topped with strawberries and flaxseeds

Lunch

- Lentil soup with a side of mixed vegetables

Dinner

- Avocado, cucumber, and tomato salad

Snacks

- Carrot sticks
- Hummus

Day 3

Breakfast

- Green smoothie (spinach, banana, almond milk)

Lunch

- Honey chicken and avocado salad

Dinner

- Baked mackerel with a side of sweet potato and kale salad

Snacks

- Walnuts
- Orange

Day 4

Breakfast

- Veggie Omelet

Lunch

- Chickpea salad with mixed greens, cucumber, and olive oil dressing

Dinner

- Baked almond chicken with cherry and balsamic

Snacks

- Celery sticks
- Hummus

Day 5

Breakfast

- Blueberry flax smoothie

Lunch

- Grilled chicken and mushrooms

Dinner

- Baked tofu with a side of brown rice and roasted Brussels sprouts

Snacks

- Apple
- Almonds

Day 6

Breakfast

- Energy oats

Lunch

- Fresh cucumber salad

Dinner

- Baked salmon with garlic and dijon dressing

Snacks

- Carrot sticks
- Hummus

Day 7

Breakfast

- Mediterranean breakfast

Lunch

- One-pot beans and zucchini penne

Dinner

- Baked tuna and asparagus

Snacks

- Celery sticks
- Hummus

Remember to drink plenty of water throughout the day, and feel free to adjust this plan to suit your taste preferences and dietary needs. It's always a good idea to consult with a healthcare professional or dietitian when making significant changes to your diet.

Sample Recipes

With the meal plan outlined in the previous chapter, here are a few sample recipes to get you started on your journey to healthier eating.

Baked Mackerel with Sweet Potato and Kale Salad

Ingredients:

- 4 mackerel fillets
- 2 sweet potatoes, peeled and cubed
- 1 bunch of kale, chopped
- 2 tablespoons olive oil
- 1 tablespoon lemon juice
- Salt and pepper to taste

Instructions:

1. Preheat your oven to 375°F (190°C).
2. In a large bowl, toss the cubed sweet potatoes with 1 tablespoon of olive oil and season with salt and pepper.
3. Place the sweet potatoes on a baking sheet and roast in the oven for 25 minutes, or until tender.
4. While the sweet potatoes are roasting, season the mackerel fillets with salt and pepper and place them on a separate baking sheet.
5. Bake the mackerel fillets in the oven for 10-12 minutes, or until flaky and cooked through.
6. In a bowl, mix the chopped kale, lemon juice, and remaining tablespoon of olive oil.

7. Once the sweet potatoes are done roasting, add them to the bowl with the kale and toss to combine.
8. Serve the baked mackerel fillets on a bed of sweet potato and kale salad.

Salmon Steak and Cauliflower Mash

Ingredients:

For the steak:

- 5 ounces Salmon steak
- Salt, to taste
- Pepper, to taste
- ¼ lemon
- For the Mash
- 1 large Cauliflower
- 2 tablespoons Silken tofu
- 1 teaspoon Lemon juice
- ½ teaspoon Garlic powder
- Salt, to taste
- Pepper, to taste
- Pinch of nutmeg

Instructions:

1. Grill salmon in a skillet on medium-high heat. Allow 2 minutes per side. Sprinkle with salt and pepper before turning, then sprinkle with salt and pepper again.
2. Arrange on a plate and squeeze lemon juice on top. Set aside.
3. Cut the cauliflower into florets.
4. If you have a steamer, steam florets until tender but not wilted. Alternatively, you can boil the florets in salted water until just tender. Set aside.

5. In a separate small bowl, mix tofu, lemon juice, garlic powder, salt, pepper, and nutmeg. Consistency should be smooth, with a few tofu grains – like cream cheese.
6. Using a blender, pulse the cauliflower until the consistency is okay with you. You can go smooth or with a few chunks. Spoon into a bowl and top with tofu dressing.
7. Serve grilled salmon steak with cauliflower mash.

Avocado, Cucumber, and Tomato Salad

Ingredients:

- 1/4 cup Extra-virgin olive oil
- 1 piece Lemon, juiced
- 1/4 teaspoon Cumin, ground
- Salt to taste
- Freshly ground black pepper to taste
- 3 medium Avocados, cubed
- 1 pint cherry tomatoes halved
- 1 small cucumber, sliced into half-moons
- 1/3 cup Corn
- 1 piece Jalepeño, minced (optional)
- 2 tablespoons Cilantro, chopped

Instructions:

1. In a small bowl, whisk together the extra-virgin olive oil, the juice from one lemon, ground cumin, salt, and freshly ground black pepper to create your dressing. Set aside.
2. In a large salad bowl, add the cubed avocados, halved cherry tomatoes, sliced cucumber, and corn.
3. If you're adding heat to the salad, finely mince your jalapeño and add it to the salad bowl.
4. Pour the dressing over the salad ingredients. Toss gently until all ingredients are well coated in the dressing.

5. Sprinkle chopped cilantro over the salad for an extra burst of flavor.
6. For the best taste, let the salad sit for about 10 minutes before serving to allow the flavors to meld together.
7. Serve immediately. This salad is a refreshing side dish or can also be enjoyed as a light main course.

Honey Chicken and Avocado Salad

Ingredients:

- 4 deboned chicken thighs
- 1 full head of chopped Romaine lettuce
- 1/2 cup of cherry tomatoes, sliced in two
- 1/2 of a thinly sliced red onion
- 2 cubed avocados

For the marinade:

- 1 spoonful of honey
- A dash of chili powder, about 1/2 teaspoon
- 2 minced cloves of garlic
- 4 spoonfuls of lime juice
- 1 small jalapeño pepper, finely chopped
- A sprinkle of salt, about 1 teaspoon
- 1 tablespoon of olive oil

For the dressing:

- 4 tablespoons of juice from a lime
- 2 tablespoons of honey
- A teaspoon of salt
- 4 tablespoons of olive oil
- Half a teaspoon of pepper

Instructions:

1. In a bowl of medium size, mix together all the ingredients for the chicken marinade.
2. Toss in the chicken thighs and marinate for at least one hour.
3. Use a cast-iron frying pan to prepare the chicken over high heat until it develops a pleasing sear on its surface and is no longer pink inside, which should take about four minutes per side. Afterward, remove the chicken and set it aside.
4. Put the cut lettuce, tomatoes, red onion, and avocados into a big salad bowl.
5. Cut the prepared chicken thighs into pieces and incorporate them into the salad bowl.
6. Gather all the dressing ingredients and mix them together in a small bowl.
7. Toss the salad with the dressing and serve immediately.

Veggie Omelet

Ingredients:

- 4 teaspoons Extra-virgin olive oil
- 1 small Onion, chopped fine
- 4 pieces (about 1 1/2cups) Plum tomatoes, chopped fine
- 10 ounces Spinach, chopped
- Salt to taste
- Black pepper, freshly ground, to taste
- 12 pieces of Egg whites
- 2 tablespoons Water
- Non-stick cooking spray

Instructions:

1. In a small skillet, heat the oil over medium heat. Add the onions, tomatoes, spinach, and a pinch of salt. Cook until the onion is soft, about 3 to 5 minutes.
2. Add pepper, to taste, and another pinch of salt. Cook for another minute.
3. Remove the spinach mixture from the heat to a bowl. Cover and keep warm.
4. In a bowl of medium size, beat the egg whites, water, and a small amount of salt and pepper until it forms a frothy mixture.

5. Gently apply cooking spray to a medium-sized nonstick frying pan or omelet pan and warm it over a medium flame.
6. Pour in 1/4 of the egg whites, making sure to spread them evenly across the base of the pan. Allow them to cook until they firm up, which should take about 1.5 to 2 minutes.
7. With a rubber spatula, lift the cooked portion of the eggs allowing the liquid egg to flow beneath it. Place 1/4 of the spinach mixture over one half of the omelet, fold it in half, and gently transfer it onto a serving dish.
8. Repeat with the remaining egg whites and spinach mixture. Serve.

Baked Almond Chicken with Cherry and Balsamic

Ingredients:

For the chicken:

- 1 pound chicken breasts, either pounded thin or thinly sliced
- 1/4 cup Greek yogurt, plain
- Pepper, to taste
- 1/2 teaspoon Kosher salt
- 1 1/4 cup Almonds, slivered

For the sauce:

- 1 teaspoon Cooking oil
- 1/2 cup Red onion, chopped
- 1/4 teaspoon Kosher salt
- 1 1/2 teaspoon fresh thyme, minced
- Pepper, to taste
- 3 tablespoons Balsamic vinegar
- 1/2 cup cherry preserves

Instructions:

1. Preheat oven to 350°F. Line a baking sheet with foil and spritz with nonstick spray.
2. Mix Greek yogurt, pepper, and salt in a bowl.
3. Add chicken. Mix until the chicken is fully coated.
4. Place almonds on a baking sheet or a shallow dish.

5. Coat the marinated chicken with the almonds. Coat both sides. Place coated chicken breasts on a lined baking sheet.
6. Bake chicken for 15-20 minutes, or until golden brown and cooked through.
7. While the chicken is baking, heat oil in a saucepan.
8. On medium heat, saute onion until soft and translucent.
9. Add thyme, salt, and pepper. Saute for another minute.
10. Add cherry preserves and vinegar. Stir until preserves melt into the sauce.
11. Serve sauce over chicken.

Blueberry Flax Smoothie

Ingredients:

- 1 cup blueberries, frozen
- 1 tablespoon flaxseed, ground
- A handful of spinach leaves
- 1/4 cup full-fat Greek yogurt (you can use any flavored yogurt you want)
- 1 cup coconut milk OR any kind of milk

Instructions:

1. Start by adding the coconut milk (or your choice of milk) into the blender. Adding the liquid first will help your blender run more efficiently.
2. Next, add in the frozen blueberries, ground flaxseed, and spinach leaves.
3. Scoop in the full-fat Greek yogurt. This will give your smoothie a creamy texture and a boost of protein.
4. Secure the lid on the blender and blend on high until all the ingredients are well combined and the smoothie is creamy. This usually takes around 1-2 minutes.
5. Once blended, taste the smoothie and adjust as needed. You may want to add a little honey or sweetener if you prefer it sweeter, or more milk if you want a thinner consistency.
6. Pour the smoothie into a glass or travel cup and enjoy immediately for the best taste and consistency.

Grilled Chicken and Mushrooms

Ingredients:

- 4 pieces of chicken breasts, boneless and skinless
- 3 cups baby spinach
- 2 cups Mushrooms, sliced
- 3 stalks Green onions, sliced
- 2 tablespoons Pecans, chopped
- 2 teaspoons smoked paprika
- 1 teaspoon Onion powder
- ½ teaspoon Garlic powder
- 1 teaspoon dried thyme
- Cooking oil
- Sea salt and freshly ground black pepper, to taste

Instructions:

1. Preheat your grill to medium-high heat.
2. Combine the paprika, onion powder, garlic powder, and dried thyme in a small bowl. Season with salt and pepper.
3. Sprinkle the chicken with the seasoning mix.
4. Grill the chicken for 10 to 15 minutes per side on the preheated grill.

5. Swirl cooking oil in a large skillet and sauté the spinach, mushrooms, onions, and pecans until the mushrooms are tender. Set aside and keep warm.
6. Top each chicken breast with the spinach mixture to serve.

Energy Oats

Ingredients:

- 1 cup Rolled oats
- 1 tablespoon Walnuts
- 1 tablespoon Flaxseed
- 1 tablespoon Almonds, sliced
- 1 cup Blueberries OR fruit of choice
- 1 cup Almond OR soy milk

Instructions:

1. Start by placing the rolled oats in a bowl or mason jar if you prefer overnight oats.
2. Pour over the almond milk or soy milk, ensuring the oats are fully submerged. Stir well to combine.
3. Next, add the walnuts, flaxseed, and sliced almonds to the mixture. Stir again to evenly distribute the nuts and seeds throughout the oats.
4. If you're preparing this for overnight oats, cover the bowl or jar and place it in the refrigerator. Let it sit overnight or for at least 6 hours. This allows the oats to absorb the milk and soften.
5. In the morning or after the soaking period, give the oats a good stir. You may need to add a little more milk to reach your desired consistency.

6. Top the oats with blueberries or fruit of your choice. If you're using a jar, you can layer the fruits and oats for a visually appealing breakfast.
7. Enjoy your Energy Oats as they are or warm them up slightly in the microwave if you prefer.

Fresh Cucumber Salad

Ingredients:

- 1 large English cucumber, halved and sliced
- 2 cups Grape tomatoes, halved
- 1 medium Red onion, halved and thinly sliced
- 1/2 cup Balsamic vinaigrette
- 3/4 cup Reduced-fat feta cheese, crumbled

Instructions:

1. Begin by preparing your vegetables. Halve the English cucumber lengthwise and then slice it into thin half-moons. Halve the grape tomatoes and set them aside. Finally, halve the red onion and slice it thinly.
2. In a large salad bowl, combine the sliced cucumber, halved tomatoes, and thinly sliced red onion.
3. Pour the balsamic vinaigrette over the vegetables in the bowl. Gently toss until all the vegetables are well coated with the vinaigrette.
4. Crumble the reduced-fat feta cheese over the top of the salad.
5. For optimal flavor, let the salad sit for about 15 minutes before serving to allow the flavors to meld together.
6. Serve the Fresh Cucumber Salad as a refreshing side dish or enjoy it as a light, healthy meal on its own.

Baked Salmon with Garlic and Dijon Dressing

Ingredients:

- 1 1/2 pound salmon filet
- 2 tablespoons fresh parsley, chopped
- 2 tablespoons light olive oil
- 2 tablespoons fresh lemon juice
- 3 Garlic cloves, pressed
- 1/2 tablespoon Dijon mustard
- 1/2 teaspoon Sea salt
- 1/8 teaspoon Black pepper
- 1/2 Lemon, sliced into 4 rings

Instructions:

1. Set your oven to preheat at 450°F and prepare a rimmed baking tray by lining it with either a Silpat or aluminum foil.
2. Divide the salmon into 4 pieces and position them on the prepared baking tray with the skin side facing down.
3. In a small bowl, mix together the parsley, garlic, oil, lemon juice, Dijon, salt, and pepper. Apply this mixture liberally over the top and sides of the salmon pieces, then garnish each portion with a slice of lemon.
4. Bake at 450°F for 12-15 min or until just cooked through and flaky. Don't overcook.

Mediterranean Breakfast

Ingredients:

- 2 Eggs, either poached or hard-boiled
- 1/2 medium avocado, diced
- 1 cup Tomato, diced
- 1 cup Cucumber, diced
- Parsley, chopped, for garnish

Instructions:

1. To prepare your eggs, start by poaching them or making them hard-boiled. For poached eggs, gently slide cracked eggs into simmering water and cook for 3-4 minutes for a runny yolk or longer for a firmer yolk. Use a slotted spoon to carefully remove and drain on a paper towel. For hard-boiled eggs, boil them in water for 9-12 minutes, then drain and cool in ice water before peeling.
2. While the eggs are cooking, dice the avocado, tomato, and cucumber into bite-sized pieces.
3. Arrange the diced avocado, tomato, and cucumber on a plate or in a bowl.
4. Once the eggs are cooked to your liking, add them to the plate or bowl with the diced vegetables.

5. Garnish the dish with chopped parsley for a burst of fresh flavor
6. Serve your Mediterranean Breakfast as is, or with a slice of whole-grain toast for added fiber.

One-pot beans and Zucchini Penne

Ingredients:

- 8 ounces of Dry penne
- 1/4 cup Onion, diced
- 1/4 cup Water
- 3 cloves Garlic, pressed
- 1 tablespoon dried oregano
- 1 tablespoon dried basil
- 3 Zucchinis, cubed
- 2 cans Great Northern beans, rinsed and drained
- 2 28-ounce cans of diced tomatoes
- Sea salt and ground pepper, to taste

Instructions:

1. Start by preparing your vegetables: dice the onion, press the garlic, and cube the zucchini.
2. In a large pot, sauté the diced onion in 1/4 cup of water until it becomes translucent.
3. Add the pressed garlic to the pot and continue to sauté until it is fragrant.
4. Stir in the dried oregano and dried basil to the pot, allowing the flavors to meld together for about a minute.
5. Add the cubed zucchinis to the pot and stir everything together, making sure the zucchinis are well-coated with the onion, garlic, and herb mixture.

6. Rinely rinse and drain the Great Northern beans, then add them to the pot.
7. Pour the two 28-ounce cans of diced tomatoes (including the juice) into the pot.
8. Season the mixture with sea salt and ground pepper, adjusting to taste.
9. Let the mixture come to a simmer and allow it to cook for about 10 minutes, or until the zucchini becomes tender.
10. While the mixture is simmering, cook the dry penne according to the package instructions until it is al dente.
11. Once the penne is cooked, drain it and add it to the pot, stirring everything together until the pasta is well-coated with the tomato and vegetable mixture.
12. Allow the pasta to simmer in the pot for a few more minutes so it can absorb some of the flavors
13. Serve your One-pot Beans and Zucchini Penne hot, garnished with fresh basil or a sprinkle of parmesan cheese if desired.

Baked Tuna and Asparagus

Ingredients:

- 2 5-ounce tuna fillets
- 14 ounces Young potatoes
- 8 Asparagus spears, trimmed and halved
- 2 handfuls cherry tomatoes
- 1 handful fresh basil leaves
- 2 tablespoons Extra-virgin olive oil
- 1 tablespoon Balsamic vinegar

Instructions:

1. Preheat your oven to 400°F (200°C).
2. In a large pot of boiling salted water, cook the potatoes for about 10 minutes until they are just tender. Add the asparagus in the last 3 minutes of cooking. Drain and set aside.
3. Take a large piece of parchment paper or foil and place the potatoes, asparagus, and cherry tomatoes in the center. Top with the tuna fillets.
4. In a small bowl, whisk together the extra-virgin olive oil and balsamic vinegar. Drizzle this mixture over the tuna and vegetables. Season with salt and pepper.
5. Fold the parchment or foil around the ingredients to form a sealed packet.

6. Bake in the preheated oven for 15-20 minutes, or until the tuna is cooked to your liking.
7. Remove from the oven and carefully open the packet, allowing the steam to escape. Sprinkle the fresh basil leaves on top before serving.

Avocado Spinach Smoothie

Ingredients:

- 1 ripe avocado
- 2 cups of fresh spinach
- 1 ripe banana
- 1 cup of almond milk (or any other non-dairy milk)
- A handful of ice cubes

Instructions:

1. Cut the avocado in half and remove the pit. Scoop out the flesh and put it in a blender.
2. Add the spinach to the blender. If using a smaller blender, you might need to add the spinach in batches.
3. Peel the banana and add it to the blender.
4. Pour the almond milk into the blender.
5. Add the ice cubes.
6. Blend on high speed until all ingredients are well combined and the smoothie is creamy and smooth.
7. Taste the smoothie and adjust as necessary. You might want to add a bit more almond milk if it's too thick, or a bit more banana if you want it sweeter.
8. Pour into a glass and enjoy your nutritious and delicious Avocado Spinach Smoothie!

Quinoa Salad with Salmon and Veggies

Ingredients:

- 1 cup cooked quinoa
- 1 grilled salmon fillet
- 1 cup of mixed vegetables (like bell peppers, cucumbers, and cherry tomatoes)
- A squeeze of lemon juice
- Olive oil
- Salt and pepper to taste

Instructions:

1. Start by cooking your quinoa according to the package instructions. Once cooked, set it aside to cool.
2. Grill your salmon fillet. You can season it with a little salt, pepper, and lemon juice before grilling. Once it's cooked to your liking, flake the salmon with a fork.
3. Chop your mixed vegetables into bite-sized pieces. You can use any veggies you like, but colorful bell peppers, crunchy cucumbers, and sweet cherry tomatoes work well.
4. In a large bowl, combine the cooled quinoa, flaked salmon, and chopped veggies.
5. Drizzle the salad with olive oil and a squeeze of fresh lemon juice. Season with salt and pepper to taste, then toss everything together until well combined.

6. Your Quinoa Salad with Salmon and Veggies is ready to serve! It makes a great lunch or dinner, and the leftovers are perfect for a quick and healthy meal.

Sweet Potato and Black Bean Tacos

Ingredients:

- 2 medium sweet potatoes
- 1 can black beans, rinsed and drained
- Whole grain tortillas
- Salsa of your choice
- Lettuce
- 1 ripe avocado
- Olive oil, salt, and pepper for seasoning

Instructions:

1. Preheat your oven to 400°F (200°C). Peel the sweet potatoes and cut them into bite-sized chunks. Place them on a baking sheet, drizzle with olive oil, sprinkle with salt and pepper, and toss to coat. Roast in the oven for about 20-25 minutes or until they are tender and lightly browned.
2. While the sweet potatoes are roasting, heat the black beans in a small saucepan over medium heat. You can add a little bit of salt and pepper for flavor if you'd like.
3. Warm the whole grain tortillas in a dry skillet over medium heat, just until they're pliable.
4. To assemble the tacos, spread a layer of black beans on each tortilla. Top with roasted sweet potatoes. Add a

few pieces of lettuce, a spoonful of salsa, and some slices of avocado.
5. Fold the tortillas over and enjoy your Sweet Potato and Black Bean Tacos while warm!

Blueberry Almond Overnight Oats

Ingredients:

- 1/2 cup of oats
- 1/2 cup of almond milk
- 1/2 cup of fresh blueberries
- 1 tablespoon of honey or sweetener of choice
- 2 tablespoons of almond butter
- Optional toppings: extra blueberries, sliced almonds, chia seeds, etc.

Instructions:

1. In a mason jar or bowl, add the oats and almond milk. Stir until the oats are fully immersed in the milk.
2. Add the almond butter and honey (or other sweetener) to the oat and milk mixture. Stir well to combine.
3. Top with fresh blueberries and any additional toppings you'd like.
4. Cover the jar or bowl and place it in the refrigerator overnight (or for at least 6 hours).
5. In the morning, give the oats a good stir. You may need to add a bit more almond milk if the mixture is too thick.
6. Enjoy your Blueberry Almond Overnight Oats cold straight from the fridge, or warm it up if you prefer!

Green Tea Matcha Smoothie

Ingredients:

- 1 teaspoon of matcha green tea powder
- 1 banana
- 1 cup of unsweetened almond milk (or any other milk of your choice)
- 1 handful of spinach
- 1 tablespoon of honey or sweetener of choice
- Ice cubes

Instructions:

1. In a blender, add the almond milk and matcha green tea powder. Blend until the matcha is fully dissolved.
2. Add the banana, spinach, and honey (or other sweetener) to the blender.
3. Fill the blender with ice cubes to the desired level. The more ice you add, the thicker your smoothie will be.
4. Blend all the ingredients until smooth and creamy.
5. Pour the smoothie into a glass and enjoy!

Turmeric and Ginger Stir-Fry

Ingredients:

- 2 tablespoons of olive oil
- 1 tablespoon of freshly grated ginger
- 2 cloves of garlic, minced
- 1 teaspoon of turmeric powder
- 1 bell pepper, sliced
- 1 onion, sliced
- 2 medium carrots, julienned
- 1 zucchini, sliced
- Salt and pepper to taste
- Soy sauce or tamari for serving (optional)
- Fresh cilantro for garnish (optional)

Instructions:

1. Heat the olive oil in a large skillet or wok over medium heat.
2. Add the ginger and garlic to the skillet and stir-fry for about 30 seconds until fragrant.
3. Add the turmeric powder to the skillet and stir to combine with the ginger and garlic.
4. Add the bell pepper, onion, carrots, and zucchini to the skillet. Season with salt and pepper to taste.
5. Stir-fry the vegetables for about 5-7 minutes, or until they are tender-crisp.

6. If desired, you can add a splash of soy sauce or tamari for extra flavor. Stir well to ensure all the vegetables are coated.
7. Remove from heat and garnish with fresh cilantro, if using.
8. Serve your Turmeric and Ginger Stir-Fry warm with a side of brown rice or quinoa, if desired!

Conclusion

Congratulations on reaching the end of this comprehensive Acne Diet Guide! Your dedication to understanding and managing your acne through diet and nutrition is commendable. This journey towards healthier skin can be challenging, but by taking the time to read this guide, you've already taken a significant stride towards achieving your goals.

Throughout this guide, we've navigated through the complex relationship between diet and acne. We've identified foods that can potentially trigger acne, discussed how to plan an acne-friendly diet, and emphasized the importance of monitoring your progress. Each of these steps is a cornerstone in establishing a dietary routine that can help combat acne.

Remember, knowledge is your most powerful weapon in this battle against acne. Now, you are armed with a deeper understanding of how certain foods can influence your skin's health. This newfound knowledge can guide you in making informed decisions about your diet, helping you choose foods that nourish your body and your skin.

The acne diet isn't about deprivation; it's about making smart food choices based on knowledge and understanding. It's recognizing that the food you consume can have a direct impact on the health and appearance of your skin. It's about finding a balance between enjoying the foods you love and feeding your body the nutrients it needs to fight acne.

As you embark on this journey, remember that every individual's body reacts differently to different foods. The acne diet is not a one-size-fits-all solution but rather a guideline that can be personalized to fit your unique needs and lifestyle. You may find that some foods work better for you than others, and that's perfectly fine. The goal is to find what works best for you.

While diet plays a crucial role in managing acne, it's important to remember that it's not the only factor. Genetics, hormones, stress levels, and your skincare regime also contribute to your skin's health. Therefore, adopting an acne-friendly diet should complement other aspects of a comprehensive acne management plan.

Patience, perseverance, and consistency are key. Changes in skin health aren't always immediate, but every small step you take brings you closer to your goal. And remember, it's not about achieving flawless skin overnight, but about improving and maintaining your skin health over time.

Don't hesitate to seek professional help if needed. Dermatologists and dietitians can provide personalized advice and guidance, particularly if you're dealing with persistent or severe acne. They can help identify any other potential triggers or underlying issues that may be contributing to your acne.

By reaching this point, you've demonstrated a commitment to managing your acne in a holistic and sustainable way. The road ahead may have its challenges, but every change you make is a testament to your resilience and dedication.

In conclusion, the journey towards clearer, healthier skin begins from within - from the foods you consume to the lifestyle choices you make. Remember, you're not alone in this journey. Acne is a common condition, and many individuals are walking similar paths toward better skin health.

So, let's celebrate your progress so far and look forward to the journey ahead. Here's to making informed choices, to patience and persistence, and most importantly, to healthier, happier skin. You are now well-equipped with the knowledge and tools to take control of your skin health. Keep going, your efforts will pay off.

Thank you once again for choosing this guide as part of your journey towards healthier skin. Congratulations on completing this guide, and good luck on your path to clearer, healthier skin!

FAQ

What is acne?

Acne is a common skin condition that occurs when hair follicles under the skin become clogged with oil and dead skin cells. It can cause various types of skin blemishes, including blackheads, whiteheads, pimples, and cysts.

How does diet affect acne?

While diet alone cannot cause or cure acne, it can influence the severity and frequency of breakouts. Certain foods, especially those high in refined sugars and dairy, can trigger inflammation and hormonal fluctuations that contribute to acne.

What is an acne diet?

An acne diet is a way of eating that aims to reduce inflammation and balance hormones in the body to help manage acne. It typically involves consuming more fruits, vegetables, lean proteins, and whole grains, while limiting intake of processed foods, sugars, and dairy.

Which foods should I avoid on an acne diet?

While everyone's body responds differently, common acne-triggering foods include dairy products, sugary foods and drinks, fast food, and foods high in refined carbohydrates like white bread and pasta.

Are there any foods that help fight acne?

Yes, foods rich in antioxidants, omega-3 fatty acids, and zinc can help fight acne. Examples include berries, oranges, salmon, almonds, and pumpkin seeds. Drinking plenty of water and green tea can also help flush out toxins and reduce inflammation.

How long does it take for dietary changes to affect acne?

It can take several weeks to a few months to see improvements in your skin after making dietary changes. This is because skin regeneration takes time, and the effects of dietary changes on the body need time to manifest in the skin.

What should I do if my acne doesn't improve after changing my diet?

If your acne doesn't improve after several months of following an acne diet, it might be time to consult a dermatologist or a dietitian. They can provide personalized advice and help identify any other potential triggers or underlying issues that may be contributing to your acne.

References and Helpful Links

Harris, S. (2018, July 31). Can dietary changes help acne? https://www.medicalnewstoday.com/articles/322639

Migala, J. (2018, August 9). 8 diet tips for preventing acne. EverydayHealth.com. https://www.everydayhealth.com/acne-pictures/acne-diet-dos-and-donts.aspx

Cirino, E. (2023, February 14). Anti-Acne diet. Healthline. https://www.healthline.com/health/anti-acne-diet

Harris, S. (2018b, July 31). Can dietary changes help acne? https://www.medicalnewstoday.com/articles/32263

Acne management | DermNet. (n.d.). https://dermnetnz.org/topics/acne-treatment

Burke, D. (2023, June 26). Everything you want to know about acne. Healthline. https://www.healthline.com/health/skin/acne

Acne - Symptoms and causes - Mayo Clinic. (2022, October 8). Mayo Clinic. https://www.mayoclinic.org/diseases-conditions/acne/symptoms-causes/syc-20368047f

Can the right diet get rid of acne? (n.d.). https://www.aad.org. https://www.aad.org/public/diseases/acne/causes/diet

Pappas, A. (2009). The relationship of diet and acne: A review. Dermato-Endocrinology, 1(5), 262–267. https://www.ncbi.nlm.nih.gov/pmc/articles/PMC2836431/

www.ingramcontent.com/pod-product-compliance
Lightning Source LLC
LaVergne TN
LVHW012033060526
838201LV00061B/4590